Glossary

AIDS: acquired immune deficiency syndrome

AZT: azidothymidine, an antiretroviral drug, also known as zidovudine

CCR5: chemokine co-receptor expressed by cells susceptible to HIV infection

CDC classification system: Centers for Disease Control (Atlanta, USA) staging classification for HIV disease

CD4 molecule: receptor expressed by cells susceptible to HIV infection. Numbers of CD4-positive lymphocytes decline with increasing immunosuppression

CIN: cervical intraepithelial neoplasia, also known as squamous intraepithelial lesion

Co-trimoxazole: trimethoprim–sulfamethoxazole, commonly used as prophylaxis against *Pneumocystis carinii* pneumonia

CXCR4: chemokine co-receptor expressed by cells susceptible to HIV infection

ddC: zalcitabine, an antiretroviral drug

ddI: didanosine, an antiretroviral drug

d4T: stavudine, an antiretroviral drug

HAART: highly active antiretroviral therapy, a combination of three or more antiretroviral drugs

HIV: human immunodeficiency virus

HPV: human papillomavirus

HSV: herpes simplex virus

IVDU: intravenous drug user

NA: nucleoside analog, a class of antiretroviral drug, also known as nucleoside reverse transcriptase inhibitor

NNRTI: non-nucleoside reverse transcriptase inhibitor, a class of antiretroviral drug

Plasma HIV viral load: a quantitative assessment of the amount of HIV in the blood indicating the rate of viral replication and usually expressed as the number of HIV viral RNA copies per ml of plasma

p24Ag: HIV core antigen

PCP: *Pneumocystis carinii* pneumonia, an AIDS-defining illness

PI: protease inhibitor, a class of antiretroviral drug

PID: pelvic inflammatory disease

STI: sexually transmitted infection

SIL: squamous intraepithelial lesion, also known as cervical intraepithelial neoplasia or CIN

3TC: lamivudine, an antiretroviral drug

FAST FACTS

HIV in Obstetrics and Gynecology

Indispensable

Guides to

Clinical

Practice

HIV in Obstetrics and Gynaecology
A0039363

Oxford

Fast Facts – HIV in Obstetrics and Gynecology
First published May 2001

Text © 2001 J Richard Smith, Naomi Low-Beer, Bruce A Barron
© 2001 in this edition Health Press Limited
Queen Street, Abingdon, Oxford OX14 3JR, UK
Tel: +44 (0)1235 523233
Fax: +44 (0)1235 523238

Fast Facts is a trade mark of Health Press Limited.

A CIP catalog record for this title is available from the British Library.

ISBN 1-899541-61-6

Smith, JR (Richard)
Fast Facts – HIV in Obstetrics and Gynecology/
J Richard Smith, Naomi Low-Beer, Bruce A Barron

Printed by Fine Print (Services) Ltd, Oxford, UK.

Introduction

In 1981, five cases of *Pneumocystis carinii* pneumonia (PCP) in previously healthy homosexual men from the Los Angeles area were reported to the United States Centers for Disease Control (CDC) in Atlanta, Georgia. Shortly thereafter, reports from New York described PCP and Kaposi's sarcoma in homosexual men. The reports suggested an underlying deficiency in cell-mediated immunity, and the condition was called 'acquired immune deficiency syndrome' (AIDS). Initially, the only apparent link was homosexual behavior. However, over the next 2 years similar cases were recognized among hemophiliacs, intravenous drug users (IVDUs), blood transfusion recipients and heterosexuals (male and female). Later, children born to HIV-infected mothers were also shown to be at risk.

In Paris in 1983, the causative virus was discovered in a patient with lymphadenopathy. It was termed 'lymphadenopathy-associated virus' (LAV). Observation of the virus was confirmed, and extended to the USA where the virus was called 'human T lymphotrophic virus type III' (HTLV III). The name 'human immunodeficiency virus' (HIV) was reached as a compromise.

Throughout the world, over 33.6 million people are estimated to be living with HIV, of whom 95% live in developing countries (Figure 1).

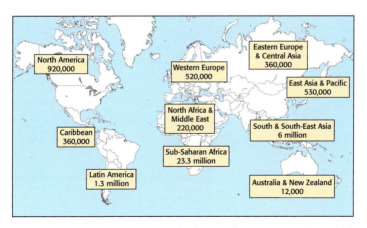

Figure 1 Adults and children estimated to be living with HIV/AIDS at the end of 1999. Data from the Joint United Nations Programme on HIV/AIDS and World Health Organization.

Approximately 46% of adults infected are women, but differences in routes of transmission give rise to substantial regional variation. For instance, in sub-Saharan Africa, where heterosexual transmission predominates, women represent over half of all adult HIV infections. In western Europe and the USA, where transmission is more common among male homosexuals and IVDUs, 20% of HIV-infected adults are women. However, there is evidence that the rate of heterosexual transmission has risen in the developed world over the past 5 years, and women are likely to represent an increasing proportion of those with HIV infection in these countries.

The prevalence of HIV infection in the UK is small compared with that in the USA (0.09% compared with 0.76% of those aged 15–49 years). In the UK, more than 5000 women have been infected with HIV, of whom over 1500 have progressed to AIDS. In England and Wales, the majority of women with HIV have acquired their infection through heterosexual exposure, and in most cases they or their partners originate from HIV-endemic countries, particularly sub-Saharan Africa. Although the early introduction of needle-exchange schemes throughout the UK has been successful in controlling the spread of HIV among IVDUs, contaminated needles remain the most common cause of HIV infection among women in Scotland.

In the USA, there are an estimated 160 000 HIV-infected women, and more than 100 000 cumulative cases of AIDS among women have been reported. HIV infections among women in the USA are increasingly concentrated in poorer sections of the population, and the groups with the greatest prevalence of HIV infection are IVDUs (or their partners), members of ethnic minorities (Hispanics and Afro-Americans) and immigrants from HIV-endemic countries. These women are also more likely to be wary of institutions, and may be reluctant to seek medical advice.

Potent combinations of antiretroviral drugs (highly active antiretroviral therapy or HAART) have resulted in a reduction in the incidence of AIDS and an increased life expectancy for those with AIDS in developed countries. The rate of new infections in these countries has not declined over the past decade, however, and the number of people infected with HIV is, therefore, growing. This represents an increasing challenge to healthcare professionals and government agencies.

CHAPTER 1

HIV infection

HIV is a retrovirus containing reverse transcriptase. This enzyme allows the virus to transcribe its RNA genome into DNA, which then integrates into the host cell's DNA (Figures 1.1 and 1.2). There are two strains of HIV, types 1 and 2 (HIV-1 and HIV-2). Globally, HIV-1 is responsible for most HIV infections; HIV-2 is relatively rare outside west Africa. As HIV is a highly variable virus, it has been further classified into groups M and O. The M group has a number of subtypes, known as clades.

HIV-1 infects cells expressing both a chemokine co-receptor (mainly CCR5 and/or CXCR4) and a CD4 molecule. Such target cells include T lymphocytes, monocytes, macrophages, microglial cells and dendritic cells.

Transmission

HIV infection is principally transmitted in the course of sexual intercourse, intravenous drug use or transfusion of blood or blood products. HIV has a fragile outer lipid membrane (derived from the host cell during budding), and the virus does not survive well outside the body. Sexual transmission can occur among heterosexuals through vaginal or anal intercourse, and among homosexuals through anal intercourse. Receptive oral intercourse has also been implicated as a mode of HIV transmission, but the risk is considered to be much smaller than with penile–vaginal or penile–anal contact.

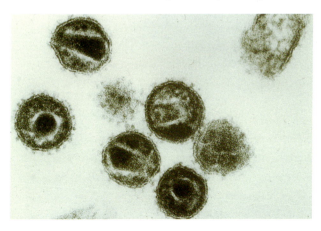

Figure 1.1
The human immunodeficiency virus.

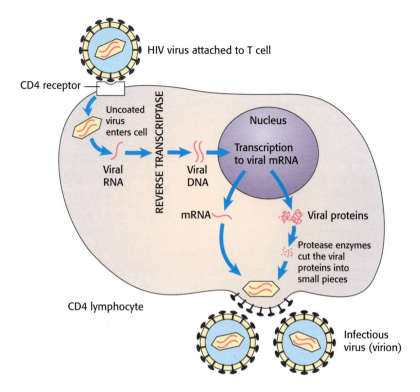

Figure 1.2 HIV entry into a CD4 lymphocyte.

Risk of sexual transmission. In European and US studies, the risk of HIV transmission per unprotected act of sexual intercourse has been estimated as 1:500–1000 for male-to-female and 1:1000–3000 for female-to-male transmission. The risk of sexual transmission depends on the degree of exposure, the infectiousness of the host and the susceptibility of the exposed individual. An elevated plasma HIV load, which is most common in those with primary HIV infection and advanced HIV disease, is the most important risk factor for transmission. It is not yet known whether reductions in viral load brought about by the use of antiretroviral therapy can reduce the rate of transmission in couples discordant for HIV infection. Other factors that increase infectivity include coexisting sexually transmitted infections (STIs) and virus type, with HIV-2 being significantly less transmissible than HIV-1. Factors increasing an individual's susceptibility to HIV infection include bacterial vaginosis and STIs.

Clinical phases

Three clinical phases follow primary HIV infection. Seroconversion occurs 2–6 weeks after infection. Levels of circulating free virus are high, and individuals may experience a glandular fever-type illness (acute seroconversion). Symptoms, when present, usually last less than 14 days. Seroconversion is followed by a prolonged clinical latency phase; during this time, viral replication continues but is controlled by host immune responses. The number of CD4-positive lymphocytes (the CD4 count) gradually falls, resulting in impaired immune function. This ultimately leads to the opportunistic infections and malignancies characteristic of AIDS. During this last phase, the plasma viral load increases and the associated decline in CD4 count accelerates.

Progression

The rate of disease progression varies considerably between individuals; without treatment, the median time from infection to AIDS development is approximately 10 years. Progression depends on a variety of host and viral factors, and is significantly altered by the use of highly active antiretroviral therapy (HAART) and prophylactic regimens. Monitoring of disease progression is by serial plasma viral load measurements and CD4 counts. The latter reflects the degree of immunosuppression, while plasma viral load indicates the rate of viral replication. The typical course of HIV infection is shown in Figure 1.3. In 1993, a revised staging classification, which combined CD4 counts and clinical information, was introduced by the CDC (Table 1.1).

HIV in women

There is no evidence that progression to AIDS or death is greater in women with HIV than in infected men receiving comparable medical care. However, women may have poorer access to healthcare facilities, which may result in delayed diagnosis and a failure to receive appropriate antiretroviral therapy or prophylaxis.

Kaposi's sarcoma, the AIDS-defining vascular tumor associated with the newly identified human herpes virus 8 (HHV8), is most commonly diagnosed in homosexual men, and is relatively rare in women. Genital tract disorders also differ between the sexes. HIV-infected women are prone to

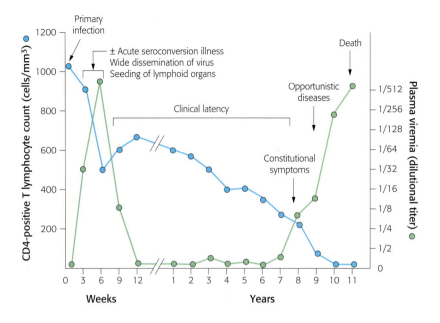

Figure 1.3 The typical course of HIV infection. Adapted from Pantaleo G *et al.* *N Engl J Med* 1993;328:327–35.

cervical neoplasia and severe vulvovaginal infection by fungal and viral agents (according to the level of immunosuppression).

Pregnancy. The effect of pregnancy on the course of HIV infection has been a subject of considerable debate. In women with advanced HIV disease, pregnancy is associated with clinical deterioration. However, women without advanced HIV disease do not appear to be at increased risk of accelerated immunosuppression during, or as a result of, pregnancy. Although mean CD4-positive lymphocyte counts decline during pregnancy, percentages of CD4-positive and CD8-positive lymphocytes remain stable throughout pregnancy and for up to 6 months postpartum.

Laboratory testing
HIV-antibody testing. HIV infection in adults is diagnosed when antibodies to HIV are detected in the blood. The standard diagnostic HIV test detects HIV-specific antibodies using enzyme-linked immunosorbent assay (ELISA)

TABLE 1.1

Revised CDC classification system for HIV disease (1993)

CD4 lymphocyte count × 10^6/liter	Clinical category		
	A	B	C
> 500	A1	B1	C1
200–500	A2	B2	C2
< 200	A3	B3	C3

Category A
- Asymptomatic HIV infection
- Persistent generalized lymphadenopathy
- Acute HIV infection

Category B (symptomatic, but not A or C)
- Bacillary angiomatosis
- Oral hairy leukoplakia
- Idiopathic thrombocytopenia purpura
- Herpes zoster
- Cervical dysplasia (moderate or severe)
- Constitutional symptoms > 1 month
- Peripheral neuropathy
- Candidiasis (oral or recurrent vaginal)
- Listeriosis
- Pelvic inflammatory disease

Category C (AIDS-defining conditions)
- Candidiasis (pulmonary or esophageal)
- Cervical cancer
- Coccidioidomycosis
- Cryptococcosis (extrapulmonary)
- Cryptosporidiosis
- Cytomegalovirus
- Herpes simplex (chronic or esophageal)
- Histoplasmosis (extrapulmonary)
- HIV-associated dementia
- HIV-associated wasting
- Isosporiasis
- Kaposi's sarcoma
- Lymphoma
- Mycobacterial infection (*Mycobacterium avium, M. kansasii, M. tuberculosis*)
- Nocardiosis
- *Pneumocystis carinii* pneumonia
- Progressive multifocal leukoencephalopathy
- Recurrent bacterial pneumonia
- Salmonellosis
- Strongyloides (extraintestinal)
- Toxoplasmosis (internal organ)

and Western blot. ELISA detects IgG antibodies to whole viral antigens, while the Western blot is used to confirm a positive ELISA (selected viral proteins are bound by HIV-specific antibody, which can then be visualized). The HIV-antibody test is 99.9% specific and sensitive when performed more than 12 weeks after HIV infection has occurred. During the 12-week 'window period', infected individuals may be antibody negative. However, due to the associated high plasma viremia, they are likely to be particularly infectious at this time.

Direct tests for the virus. The polymerase chain reaction (PCR) can be used to amplify HIV DNA from mononuclear cells in the blood, whilst reverse transcription and amplification of HIV RNA may be performed on plasma samples. These amplification techniques may be used to:
- monitor disease progression and treatment
- characterize HIV strains
- determine the presence of mutations associated with antiretroviral drug resistance
- diagnose HIV infection in infancy
- diagnose acute HIV infection during the 12-week 'window period', in which an individual may not yet test HIV-antibody positive.

Other direct tests for the virus include the p24 antigen (p24Ag) assay and viral culture, which may be used as adjuncts to amplification techniques in the diagnosis of HIV in infancy and the diagnosis of acute HIV infection.

CHAPTER 2

Managing infected women

Antiretroviral therapy

Successful treatment will achieve a sustained suppression of plasma viral load, thereby reducing the risk of AIDS-related morbidity and mortality. A summary of antiretroviral therapy treatment guidelines is shown in Table 2.1; the dosing and adverse effects associated with antiretroviral drugs are included as Appendix I. However, in practice the choice and timing of treatment is a complex and rapidly evolving area, requiring the expertise

TABLE 2.1

British HIV Association (BHIVA) guidelines for the treatment of HIV-infected adults with antiretroviral therapy, December 1999

When to initiate treatment

Presentation	Surrogate markers	Recommendation
Asymptomatic HIV infection	CD4 count > 500 cells/µl Any viral load	● Defer treatment
	CD4 count 350–500 cells/µl Viral load < 30 000 copies/ml	● Defer treatment
	CD4 count 350–500 cells/µl Viral load > 30 000 copies/ml	● Consider treatment or defer and monitor at least every 3 months
	CD4 count 0–350 cells/µl Any viral load	● Treat
Symptomatic HIV infection		● Treat

Treatment regimen

Two nucleoside analogs + protease inhibitor **or** two nucleoside analogs + two protease inhibitors **or** two nucleoside analogs + non-nucleoside reverse transcriptase inhibitor

13

TABLE 2.2

Classes of antiretroviral drugs

Nucleoside analog*

- Abacavir
- Didanosine
- Lamivudine
- Stavudine
- Zalcitabine
- Zidovudine

Protease inhibitor

- Amprenavir[†]
- Indinavir
- Nelfinavir
- Ritonavir
- Saquinavir

Non-nucleoside reverse transcriptase inhibitor

- Nevirapine
- Delavirdine[†]
- Efavirenz

*Nucleoside reverse transcriptase inhibitor
[†]Not yet licensed in Europe

of an HIV physician. Treatment should also be personalized to suit the individual needs of the patient.

Three classes of antiretroviral drug are currently used (Table 2.2):
- nucleoside analogs (NAs)
- non-nucleoside reverse transcriptase inhibitors (NNRTIs)
- protease inhibitors (PIs).

NAs and NNRTIs block the reverse transcriptase that HIV uses to transcribe RNA into DNA, thus preventing viral replication. PIs block the protease enzyme, resulting in the production of non-infectious virions.

The current standard of care is to initiate treatment with at least three antiretroviral drugs, usually two NAs plus either an NNRTI or a PI (see Table 2.1). These combination regimens, often referred to as HAART, have been widely used in developed countries since 1997. Patients should consider that their regimen will continue throughout their lives.

Consistent adherence to HAART minimizes the risk of viral resistance, which is the principal cause of treatment failure. However, patients commonly have difficulty in adhering to these regimens. This may be due to the toxic effects of the drugs (see Appendix I) and the difficulty that many patients experience in making a long-term commitment to multiple-drug therapy. Moreover, many regimens necessitate dietary restrictions and strict timing of doses.

The principles of antiretroviral therapy are similar for men and women. However, drug use during pregnancy and in women wanting to become pregnant requires special consideration, and these issues are discussed in Chapters 3 and 4, respectively.

Data on the pharmacokinetics of antiretroviral therapy in non-pregnant women are limited because of the small numbers of women recruited to HIV clinical trials. PIs can cause lipodystrophy, as they do in men, but in women this may be associated with an increase in breast tissue. The bioavailability of synthetic estrogens is significantly altered by the PIs ritonavir and nelfinavir, and by the NNRTIs efavirenz and nevirapine. This has important implications for oral contraceptive users (see pages 20–21). Teratogenicity of efavirenz has been demonstrated in animal models, and this drug should therefore be avoided in women of childbearing age who are not using effective contraception.

Prophylaxis for opportunistic infections

Pneumocystis carinii pneumonia (PCP) is the most common opportunistic infection in those with HIV disease. Indications for prophylaxis and the drug regimens used are described in Table 2.3. Non-pregnant women are managed in a similar way to men. PCP prophylaxis during pregnancy is described in Chapter 3. Other conditions for which HIV-infected patients may require prophylaxis include tuberculosis and hepatitis B. Selected patients may also benefit from prophylaxis against recurrent genital herpes simplex virus (HSV) infections and, in women, recurrent vulvovaginal candidiasis.

Cervical neoplasia

There is a strong association between HIV infection and detectable human papillomavirus (HPV) infection, and this association increases with progressive immunosuppression. Studies have demonstrated a two-fold increase in the rate of cervical intraepithelial neoplasia (CIN) and a 1.7-fold

TABLE 2.3

Prophylaxis against _Pneumocystis carinii_ infection

When to initiate

- CD4 count < 200×10^6/liter
- History of _Pneumocystis carinii_ pneumonia

Regimen

First line

- Oral co-trimoxazole, 960 mg three times weekly

Alternatives

- Oral dapsone, 50 mg daily, plus pyrimethamine, 50 mg weekly
- Inhaled nebulized pentamidine isethionate, 300 mg monthly

increase in the rate of cervical cancer in young women with HIV. Studies also suggest that CIN progresses more rapidly and is less responsive to treatment in HIV-positive women than in HIV-negative women. Invasive cervical cancer is now accepted as an AIDS-defining condition. Lower genital tract changes involving vaginal, vulval and perianal intraepithelial neoplasia have been shown to occur in HIV-positive women.

Surveillance and management of CIN. Currently, HIV-negative women are recommended to have annual cervical cytology (Pap smears) in the USA and 3-yearly cervical cytology in the UK. For HIV-infected women in the UK, most centers advise annual cytology with or without colposcopy for those with asymptomatic HIV infection and CD4 counts above 500×10^6/liter, with more frequent assessments for those with advanced disease. In the USA, surveillance for CIN tends to be more intensive, with the American College of Obstetrics and Gynecology recommending 6-monthly cervical cytology for all women with HIV infection.

Although CIN 1 abnormalities in HIV-seronegative women are generally monitored rather than treated, they should be treated in HIV-infected women because of the increased likelihood of rapid progression to CIN 3. All women, irrespective of HIV infection, should have CIN 2 and 3 abnormalities treated by large loop excision of the transformation zone

(LLETZ). More frequent colposcopic follow up is necessary for women with HIV, because they are more susceptible to persistent and recurrent cervical dysplasia.

In the USA, HPV typing is recommended in HIV-positive women with cytologically diagnosed CIN. Patients found to have carcinogenic HPV types, such as 16, 18, 31, 33, 35, 45, 51, 54, 56, 61 and 62, require very close surveillance.

Currently, the methods of choice for HPV screening are Hybrid Capture-II, a second-generation liquid hybridization assay that detects HPV DNA, and PCR, which uses primer systems to amplify HPV DNA. Both methods produce results categorized as high-risk HPV (of the types included above) positive or negative, and low-risk HPV (types 6, 11) positive or negative.

Sexually transmitted infections

Throughout the world, most women acquire their HIV infection through sexual contact and are therefore more likely to be co-infected with other sexually transmitted pathogens.

The presence of ulcerative genital disease (lymphogranuloma venereum, granuloma inguinale, chancroid, syphilis and genital herpes simplex infection) and non-ulcerative STI (*Neisseria gonorrhoeae* and *Chlamydia trachomatis*) is associated with increased shedding of HIV in the cervicovaginal secretions, and an increased risk of sexual transmission. These conditions also increase the risk of HIV acquisition. One large study in Mwanza, Tanzania, has demonstrated that the syndromic treatment of STIs with antibiotics can significantly reduce the incidence of HIV infection. More recently, bacterial vaginosis has been shown to be associated with an increased risk of both sexual and vertical transmission of HIV, possibly because of the relative reduction in the numbers of vaginal lactobacilli associated with this condition.

The presentation of STIs is unaffected by HIV infection *per se*. However, HIV-related immunosuppression is associated with recurrent vulvovaginal candidiasis, genital herpes, genital warts and severe infectious vulval ulceration (Figure 2.1), all of which may be resistant to treatment. Syphilis infection has been associated with unusual serological responses, and treatment failure is more common. It has been suggested that pelvic inflammatory disease (PID) is more common in women with HIV infection.

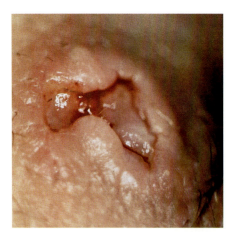

Figure 2.1 An herpetic vulval ulcer. Ulceration is particularly severe in HIV-positive women. Photograph courtesy of Dr P Greenhouse, Bristol Royal Infirmary, UK.

To some degree, this may reflect the fact that both infections are sexually transmitted. However, HIV-positive women more commonly have lower white cell counts and pyrexia on presentation. The frequency of tubo-ovarian abscesses is increased, and laparoscopic findings are commonly of greater severity than symptoms would suggest (Figure 2.2). There is no difference in the microbiology of PID in women with or without HIV infection.

Management. Sexually active HIV-infected women should be screened for STIs in a similar way to the population at large. Endocervical and urethral swabs should be analyzed for *N. gonorrhoeae* and *C. trachomatis*. Vaginal swabs for *Candida albicans*, *Trichomonas vaginalis* and bacterial vaginosis should be taken, as should a venous blood sample for *Treponema pallidum* (syphilis) serology. Careful inspection should take place for signs of genital ulceration and warts. All STIs should be treated effectively and, where possible, partners should be contacted, screened and treated in the usual way.

For those HIV-positive women suspected of having PID, a lower threshold for performing laparoscopy is warranted. This allows accurate diagnosis of PID and appropriate antibiotic therapy to be prescribed.

Menstrual disorders

High prevalences of menstrual disorders (menorrhagia, oligomenorrhea and amenorrhea) and premature menopause have been described among

HIV-positive women, but controlled studies have failed to demonstrate any clinically significant direct effect of HIV or HIV-related immunosuppression. However, coexistent substance misuse and weight loss associated with advanced HIV disease may cause amenorrhea.

A study of endocrine function showed no difference in hypothalamo-pituitary function between HIV-positive and HIV-negative women. However, a trend was seen between HIV-related immunosuppression and raised follicle-stimulating hormone (FSH) and reduced estradiol (E_2) levels, which are features of a premature menopause.

Management. Menstrual abnormalities in HIV-infected women should be managed in a similar way to uninfected women. A full gynecologic history should be taken and an abdominal and pelvic examination performed. Appropriate investigations may include an endocrine screen (FSH, LH, E_2, thyroid function tests), cervical cytology, STI screen, a pelvic ultrasound scan and endometrial sampling.

Safer sex

The male latex condom used together with a water-based lubricant throughout intercourse provides very effective protection against sexual transmission of HIV and other STIs, and they should be recommended to all couples where one individual is HIV positive and the other is HIV negative. The use of male condoms is also generally advised for HIV-positive couples

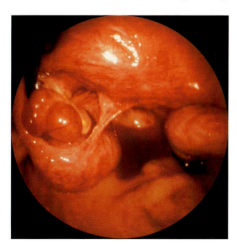

Figure 2.2 When pelvic inflammatory disease is present in an HIV-positive woman, the damage to the Fallopian tubes seen on laparoscopy is often greater than symptoms suggest. Photograph courtesy of Dr P Greenhouse, Bristol Royal Infirmary, UK.

because it reduces the risk of a partner acquiring other strains of HIV that may accelerate disease progression.

The female condom has similar contraceptive efficacy to the male condom, and it is thought that with correct use it is likely to have similar efficacy in reducing HIV transmission, although as yet there are no data to support this view. Its use has been associated with a reduction in incidence of other STIs in observational studies.

The use of other established, female-controlled barrier methods of protection, namely the cap or diaphragm, should not be advised as a means of reducing HIV transmission because they provide only partial coverage of the genital epithelium and it is not yet known whether HIV infection can occur across intact vaginal epithelium.

Spermicidal agents, such as nonoxynol-9, have been proposed as a means of preventing HIV transmission. Nonoxynol-9 inactivates HIV and other STI pathogens *in vitro*, but results of clinical trials investigating its efficacy in HIV prevention have yielded conflicting results. Moreover, when used frequently and at high doses, it has been associated with disruption of the genital epithelium, which may increase the risk of HIV transmission. The use of preparations containing nonoxynol-9 cannot therefore be recommended at present.

The dental dam has been proposed as a means of preventing HIV transmission across the female genital epithelium during oral sex. This device consists of a square piece of thin latex that is held over the vulva. There are no data available to confirm or refute this practice.

Contraception

Condoms have an associated pregnancy rate of 12% across all age groups, and many couples who do not wish to conceive choose additional methods of contraception.

The progestogen-only pill, parenteral progestogen-only contraception and sterilization have similar indications and contraindications in HIV-negative and -positive women. However, the use of the combined oral contraceptive pill may be affected by certain antiretroviral drugs; the PIs ritonavir and nelfinavir and the NNRTIs nevirapine and efavirenz affect the bioavailability of synthetic estrogens. Women taking these drugs should be advised to use alternative methods of contraception. The intrauterine contraceptive device

(IUCD) has previously been considered an unacceptable choice of contraception for HIV-positive women, principally because of concerns of an increased risk of pelvic infection and increased menstrual flow. However, more recent evidence suggests that the risk of complications associated with IUCD use is no greater in appropriately selected HIV-positive women than in their HIV-negative counterparts. The levonorgestrel intrauterine system is becoming a more popular choice of contraception in HIV-positive women because of the decreased risk of pelvic infection, high efficacy and reduced menstrual flow.

CHAPTER 3

Preconceptual care and antenatal testing

HIV-positive status known before pregnancy

Antenatal care should be non-discriminatory. All HIV-positive women should be encouraged to plan their pregnancies, and to discuss this with their physician. Dedicated preconception clinics may be an appropriate setting for this. English is not the first language of many women attending antenatal clinics, and some may be illiterate – there is an urgent need to ensure that these women are presented with appropriate information in a language that they understand; audiovisual formats may be effective.

Antiretroviral medication known to be teratogenic, such as efavirenz, should be avoided in women of childbearing age. For those considering pregnancy, non-essential medications should be discontinued, and folic acid supplements should be prescribed in the usual way for the prevention of neural tube defects. For women taking HAART, the potential carcinogenicity and teratogenicity of antiretroviral drugs should be explained. However, the practice of discontinuing HAART when planning pregnancy or when pregnancy is diagnosed, until the end of the first trimester, should not be recommended. These structured treatment interruptions or 'drug holidays' are associated with a rebound in the woman's plasma viral load, which is both hazardous to the health of the woman and may increase the risk of HIV transmission to her baby. Women planning pregnancy who continue to require prophylaxis against opportunistic infections should not discontinue their prophylaxis. Again, maintaining the woman's health must be given priority.

HIV-negative man, HIV-positive woman. If the male partner is HIV negative, artificial insemination should be considered, and the optimum time to conceive during the woman's menstrual cycle discussed.

HIV-positive man, HIV-negative woman. Couples in which the male is HIV positive and the female HIV negative may wish to have children, notwithstanding the risk associated with unprotected sexual intercourse. There are no reported cases of fathers transmitting HIV to their offspring without first infecting the mother. Some reduction in risk to the woman is possible by restricting unprotected intercourse to the time of ovulation as determined by ovulation kit or temperature chart.

The technique of 'sperm washing', whereby spermatozoa are separated from seminal plasma and non-spermatozoa cells, does reduce the risk of HIV transmission. *In-vitro* studies have demonstrated a significant reduction in both cell-free and cell-associated HIV virus in samples of spermatozoa to be used for insemination. Semprini *et al.* in Milan, Italy, have conducted a program of assisted conception for HIV-discordant couples since 1989. To date, they have reported 1902 inseminations for 605 women. This has resulted in 261 pregnancies, with no seroconversions among the women and no cases of vertical transmission. This service is now available in Milan (Italy), Barcelona (Spain), Chelsea and Westminster Hospital, London (UK) and Boston (USA).

HIV-positive man, HIV-positive woman. The use of the male condom is generally advised for HIV-positive couples because it reduces the risk of a partner acquiring other strains of HIV that might increase the speed of HIV disease progression. Although most couples are likely to choose to have unprotected sex in order to conceive, this should ideally be restricted to the periovulation phase of the woman's cycle.

Infertility. The management of infertility in a couple in which one or both partners are HIV positive poses ethical dilemmas. Sympathetic and informed counseling should be the norm, and areas for discussion include the risk of vertical transmission of HIV, the potentially adverse effect of pregnancy for women with advanced disease and the possibility of the infant being orphaned. Currently, no widely agreed guidelines exist for the management of infertility in this context. Practice will therefore depend on the individual couple, their doctor and, where involved, the local ethics committee. However, the availability of ever-improving techniques to avoid vertical transmission makes the arguments against infertility treatment less and less tenable.

HIV status unknown before pregnancy

The HIV-antibody test is highly specific and sensitive, and relatively cheap; a positive result enables measures to be taken to prevent further sexual and/or vertical transmission. Moreover, antiretroviral therapy and antibiotic prophylaxis for those with advanced HIV disease is associated with an increased life expectancy.

Antenatal testing should be offered to all women at their first clinic visit. Where there is a policy of universal antenatal HIV screening, women should be informed that the HIV test is part of routine antenatal care. If, despite adequate information, a woman chooses to decline an HIV test, her decision should be respected.

Counseling. Until recently, much emphasis was placed on extensive counseling before patients were tested for HIV infection. The current trend is to provide information succinctly. This is particularly important when information is being given in the antenatal clinic, where there is high potential for information overload. More extensive counseling should be available for those who request it (Table 3.1). Women should be aware of the importance placed on confidentiality.

A woman testing HIV-antibody positive in the antenatal clinic should be given her test result by a midwife or physician with experience and expertise

TABLE 3.1

Issues for discussion regarding diagnosis of HIV infection in pregnancy

- Vertical transmission and how its risk may be reduced (antiretroviral therapy, elective cesarean section, bottle-feeding)
- Pregnancy does not adversely affect maternal HIV disease progression, unless maternal disease is advanced
- Possible increased risk of first trimester miscarriage (see page 37), but maternal HIV infection does not otherwise affect pregnancy outcome in industrialized countries
- Timing of diagnosis of infant infection; vast majority diagnosed by 6 weeks of age, definitive diagnosis at 18 months
- Safety profile of antiretroviral drugs in pregnancy; very limited safety data except for zidovudine

in caring for HIV-positive pregnant women, and sufficient time should be available for discussion. Counseling and HIV testing should also be available for her partner.

Screening policies. Although most physicians would agree that testing for HIV infection before conception is preferable to antenatal testing, most women are not offered an HIV test until they attend an antenatal clinic. Most cases of mother-to-child transmission can be prevented if a woman is diagnosed before or during early pregnancy. Antenatal HIV testing may be implemented on a universal or a selective basis.

UK. Since 1992, the Department of Health has recommended that HIV testing, with informed consent and guaranteed confidentiality, be offered to all pregnant women in areas of high HIV prevalence (i.e. where more than 1 in 2000 live neonates is found to be infected), and selectively elsewhere to those at increased risk of HIV infection. However, the uptake of antenatal testing even in areas of relatively high prevalence, such as London, remains poor; around 70% of HIV-infected pregnant women remain undiagnosed at parturition. Despite recent advances in the prevention of vertical transmission, there continues to be a lack of awareness of the benefits of HIV testing on the part of healthcare providers – it is widely assumed that women would prefer not to find out that they have HIV infection during pregnancy. The UK is the only country in western Europe in which rates for early pediatric AIDS have not declined. Moreover, economic analyses have shown that a policy of recommending an HIV test to all pregnant women would be cost-effective, even in areas of low HIV seroprevalence. In August 1999, new national guidelines were announced which stated that all pregnant women should be offered and recommended an HIV test as an integral part of their antenatal care, irrespective of HIV seroprevalence, with the national objective of achieving an 80% reduction in mother-to-child transmission of HIV by 2002.

USA. Since 1994, the CDC has recommended that all pregnant women be offered HIV testing as part of routine early antenatal care, the proportion of HIV-infected women diagnosed through antenatal testing has greatly increased. However, although healthcare providers have been more effective in implementing these guidelines than their counterparts in the UK,

25

significant numbers of HIV-infected women in the USA receive no antenatal care; IVDUs and those from ethnic minority groups appear to be particularly neglected. Strategies to enable these women to access antenatal care could have a major impact on HIV prevention in the USA.

Advantages. A negative HIV-antibody test during pregnancy can greatly reassure many women. If the result is positive:

- the woman's infection can be managed effectively
- she can make an informed choice as to whether to continue with her pregnancy
- the risk of the child becoming infected can be greatly reduced
- the woman can make informed decisions about her future fertility
- the woman's partner can be tested, and if he is HIV seronegative, the use of condoms should prevent him from acquiring HIV infection.

Most women found to be HIV positive antenatally choose not to terminate their pregnancy. This trend is likely to continue, given the improved prognosis for those women with HIV infection and the availability of effective measures to reduce the risk of vertical transmission.

The combined interventions of prophylaxis with zidovudine (as monotherapy or in triple-agent regimens), delivery by elective cesarean section and formula feeding are associated with a reduction in mother-to-child transmission from around 25% to below 2%. The vast majority of vertically infected children are born to women whose HIV infection was not diagnosed before or during pregnancy.

Disadvantages. The main disadvantages of antenatal HIV-antibody testing relate to the psychological consequences of receiving a positive result during pregnancy. The stressful nature of this experience should not be underestimated, and counseling and support from trained professionals are required. However, it is undoubtedly more devastating for a woman to discover that she is infected only when her HIV-infected child becomes ill, and then to find out that the child's infection could probably have been prevented.

The stress of receiving a positive HIV-antibody result is likely to be compounded by fears of rejection by the woman's partner or family, and discrimination in the hospital, workplace and community as a whole. These fears highlight the need for professional support and the importance of maintaining confidentiality. A diagnosis of HIV infection can also have severe financial consequences through loss of work, the inability to gain life insurance and problems obtaining a mortgage, although these issues have improved somewhat with the introduction of HAART.

CHAPTER 4
Obstetric care

Pregnancy is only inadvisable when a woman's health is severely compromised by her HIV disease, despite treatment with HAART. The woman's already poor prognosis may be worsened by pregnancy, and the risk of transmitting HIV to her baby will be increased.

Following the decision to continue a pregnancy, the HIV-positive woman should be managed jointly by an obstetrician, HIV physician and, in the UK, a midwife. In the USA, a woman with HIV infection is considered a 'high-risk' patient and therefore not eligible for nurse/midwife care. Guidelines for the antenatal and postnatal management of HIV-positive women are shown in Table 4.1. Other agencies, such as drug-dependency units and voluntary organizations, should be involved as appropriate. Good communication between professionals is vital, and early liaison with a pediatrician should be established.

Antenatal care
Initial visit. When a woman is known to be HIV positive at her first antenatal visit, a full patient history should be taken in the usual way. A note should be made of any AIDS-defining illnesses and any antiretroviral therapy or antibiotic prophylaxis. Details of the health of any children should include whether they have been tested for HIV infection. Any history of drug misuse should be documented. Interventions to reduce the risk of mother-to-child transmission (antiretroviral therapy, cesarean section, avoidance of breastfeeding) should be discussed (see Table 4.5, page 38). A physical examination should be carried out, and investigations performed (Tables 4.2 and 4.3). These should include an STI screen and a cervical smear (if one has not been performed within the past year). Blood tests should include viral genotyping, as knowledge of the maternal genotype is important in the diagnosis of infant infection.

Follow-up visits. In addition to routine antenatal tests, 4–6-weekly CD4 counts and plasma RNA viral load measurements should be performed. For patients taking zidovudine monotherapy or combination antiretroviral

TABLE 4.1

Guidelines for the management of HIV-positive women during pregnancy and postpartum

Antepartum

Avoid:

- Cervical cerclage
- Chorionic villus sampling
- Amniocentesis
- Placental biopsy
- External cephalic version

Advise:

- Zidovudine monotherapy to reduce vertical transmission risk **or** three-drug combination antiretroviral therapy (HAART), to include zidovudine
- Oral co-trimoxazole prophylaxis if maternal CD4 count $< 200/mm^3$

Intrapartum

Avoid:

- Fetal blood sampling
- Amniotomy
- Forceps
- Fetal scalp electrodes
- Episiotomy
- Vacuum extraction

Advise:

- Early cord clamping
- Early cleansing and drying of baby
- Elective cesarean section (? bloodless) **or** planned vaginal delivery (? medical induction at term)

Postpartum

Avoid:

- Breastfeeding

Advise:

- Follow up by pediatrician for at least 18 months

TABLE 4.2

Antenatal physical examination in the HIV-positive woman

- General
  - weight
  - pallor
- Mouth and tongue
  - oral candidiasis
  - gingivitis
  - ulceration
  - oral hairy leukoplakia
  - Kaposi's sarcoma
- Lymph nodes
  - cervical
  - supraclavicular
  - axillary
  - inguinal
- Skin rashes
  - seborrheic dermatitis
  - folliculitis
  - fungal infections
  - Kaposi's sarcoma
- Nails and interdigital spaces for fungal infection
- Respiratory system
- Cardiovascular
- Abdominal/fundal palpation to check fundal height and exclude hepatosplenomegaly
- Genitals
- Inspection of the fundi for cytomegalovirus retinitis

therapy regimens, a full blood count, and urea, creatinine, electrolytes and liver function tests should be performed monthly. More frequent assessments may be necessary for those taking combination antiretroviral therapy.

Serum screening for Down's syndrome and neural tube defects should be discussed with all pregnant women. However, women with HIV should be aware that amniocentesis is associated with a theoretical risk of vertical transmission of HIV infection, rendering management of a 'high-risk' serum screening result more complex. Other invasive procedures that should be

TABLE 4.3

Antenatal clinical investigations in the HIV-positive woman

Routine tests

- Blood group
- Full blood count
- Syphilis serology
- Rubella serology
- Hepatitis B serology
- Hepatitis C serology
- Serum screening (including α-fetoprotein) for Down's syndrome and neural tube defects ± nuchal translucency scan
- Mid-stream urine sample for culture
- Cervical smear if not performed in the previous year

HIV-specific tests

- *Toxoplasma gondii* serology
- Varicella zoster serology
- Cytomegalovirus serology
- Genital infection screen for *Candida albicans,* bacterial vaginosis, *Neisseria gonorrhoeae* and *Chlamydia trachomatis*
- Blood viral genotype
- Plasma RNA viral load
- CD4 count
- Urea and electrolytes
- Liver function tests
- Confirmatory HIV test

avoided include cervical cerclage, chorionic villus sampling, cordocentesis and placental biopsy. An ultrasound scan should be performed at 18–20 weeks to detect any fetal anomaly. This is particularly important for women who have been taking potentially teratogenic drugs.

Symptoms, such as dyspnea or fatigue, which might be considered normal during pregnancy, should be interpreted with caution; they may require further investigation.

In the UK, most maternity patients hold their own notes or carry a 'shared-care' card. This may present confidentiality difficulties for HIV-positive women. Hospital physicians may offer to hold a patient's notes to improve confidentiality and, with the patient's consent, to write to their family physician. In the USA, there is currently no uniform practice.

Other aspects. Cervicovaginal infections and STIs should be detected and treated effectively during pregnancy, in view of concerns that these conditions may increase the risk of perinatal HIV transmission. Bacterial chorioamnionitis, known to be associated with vertical transmission of HIV, may predispose to or result from pre-term rupture of the membranes and/or pre-term labor. For this reason, these conditions require early intervention. In addition to antibiotics and tocolytic drugs, corticosteroids may be used when the benefit regarding fetal lung maturation outweighs the potential increase in HIV replication.

Management of HIV infection in the mother

Antiretroviral therapy. More recent advances in antiretroviral therapy have added complexity to the issue of management of HIV infection in the mother. The aim of antiretroviral therapy during pregnancy is two-fold:

- to ensure that the mother has a low, preferably 'undetectable', plasma viral RNA load during late pregnancy and at delivery, thereby minimizing the risk of vertical transmission
- to sustain this reduction in plasma viral load, thus improving and extending the length and quality of the mother's life.

Guidelines from both the USA and the UK state that pregnancy *per se* should not preclude the use of therapies of proven benefit to the mother, but that the choice and timing of treatment should take into account the possible risks to the fetus and infant.

Safety of antiretroviral therapy during pregnancy. None of the antiretroviral drugs are licensed for use in the first trimester of pregnancy, and all are classified either B or C by the US Food and Drug Administration (FDA). This indicates that their safety in human pregnancy has not been proven but the benefits of use may outweigh the risks. Perinatal exposure to zidovudine, with or without lamivudine, has been implicated in the development of mitochondrial dysfunction. The safety of zidovudine in pregnancy is discussed more fully below. Limited safety data are available for lamivudine, didanosine, nevirapine, stavudine and indinavir (Table 4.4), none of which requires any dose adjustment in pregnancy (see Appendix I). Lamivudine is usually well tolerated and readily crosses the placenta. Didanosine is commonly associated with gastrointestinal disturbances, and may occasionally cause pancreatitis. Its placental transfer is low. Nevirapine, the only NNRTI for which published pharmacokinetic data in pregnancy are available, has a long half-life of 66 hours following a single dose in pregnancy, and readily crosses the placenta. It may therefore be particularly useful for women presenting in labor who have not received prior antiretroviral therapy. A severe skin rash is the most common side-effect of treatment. Although PIs have become an integral part of combination therapy in adults and children, very limited safety data in pregnancy are available to date. Adverse effects include glucose intolerance, hyperlipidemia, lipodystrophy, renal impairment and abnormal liver function tests.

Experience of antiretroviral drugs (other than zidovudine) in pregnancy is limited, and pregnant women taking these drugs, particularly during the first trimester, must be aware of the possible risks of teratogenesis and carcinogenesis.

Initiation of antiretroviral therapy in pregnancy. The decision to initiate antiretroviral therapy for treatment of the mother should take into account plasma viral load, CD4 count and the mother's clinical state, as is the case for non-pregnant women (see Chapter 1). However, in many cases, the start of therapy may be delayed until after the first trimester. A three-drug regimen should be used, in keeping with the standard of care for non-pregnant individuals (Table 2.1, see page 13). Zidovudine is the only antiretroviral agent for which there are substantial data for safety and efficacy in pregnancy, and this agent should be incorporated into the

TABLE 4.4

Safety of antiretroviral agents in pregnancy

Drug	FDA category	Long-term animal carcinogenicity studies	Rodent teratogenicity studies
Abacavir	C	Not completed	Positive (anasarca and skeletal malformations at 1000 mg/kg [35 × human exposure] during organogenesis)
Amprenavir	C	Not completed	Positive (thymic elongation; incomplete ossification of bones; low body weight)
Delavirdine	C	Not completed	Ventricular septal defect
Didanosine	B	Negative	Negative
Efavirenz	C	Not completed	Anencephaly; anophthalmia; microphthalmia (cynomalgus monkeys)
Indinavir	C	Not completed	Negative (but extra ribs in rats)
Lamivudine	C	Negative	Negative
Nelfinavir	B	Not completed	Negative
Nevirapine	C	Not completed	Negative
Ritonavir	B	Not completed	Negative (but cryptorchidism in rats)[†]
Saquinavir	B	Not completed	Negative
Stavudine	C	Not completed	Negative (but sternal bone calcium decreases)
Zalcitabine	C	Positive in rodents (thymic lymphomas)	Positive (hydrocephalus at high dose)
Zidovudine	C	Positive in rodents at doses 12–15 times those recommended in humans (vaginal tumors)*	Positive (near lethal dose)

*No tumors observed in 734 infants exposed to antepartum zidovudine
[†]These effects seen only at maternally toxic doses

TABLE 4.4 (continued)

FDA pregnancy categories

A Adequate and well-controlled studies of pregnant women fail to demonstrate a risk to the fetus during the first trimester of pregnancy (and there is no evidence of risk during the later trimesters)

B Animal reproduction studies fail to demonstrate a risk to the fetus and adequate but well-controlled studies of pregnant women have not been conducted

C Safety in human pregnancy has not been determined, animal studies are either positive for fetal risk or have not been conducted, and the drug should not be used unless the potential benefit outweighs the potential risk to the fetus

D Positive evidence of human fetal risk based on adverse reaction data from investigational or marketing experiences, but the potential benefits from use of the drug in pregnant women may be acceptable despite its potential risks

X Studies in animals or reports of adverse reactions have indicated that the risk associated with the use of the drug in pregnant women clearly outweighs any possible benefits

chosen combination regimen unless there is a history of zidovudine resistance.

Pregnancy in women already taking antiretroviral therapy. Increasing numbers of HIV-positive women are conceiving while taking antiretroviral therapy. If their regimen does not include zidovudine, this drug should be substituted or added. Zidovudine and stavudine should not be taken concurrently because of pharmacological antagonism. Some women may wish to discontinue antiretroviral therapy prior to conception or after pregnancy is diagnosed until the end of the first trimester to reduce the risk of teratogenesis. Although most physicians would not recommend discontinuation of therapy during pregnancy, those who choose to do so should be advised to discontinue all drugs simultaneously and subsequently reintroduce them simultaneously; this minimizes the risk of drug resistance. All pregnant women currently receiving or having previously received antiretroviral therapy should be monitored for resistance mutations. For pregnant women with zidovudine-resistant virus, combination therapy with an alternative NA should be considered.

Women presenting late in pregnancy. For women presenting with HIV infection too late in pregnancy to allow formal immunologic and virologic assessment, zidovudine should be administered as quickly as possible, with the possible addition of lamivudine and nevirapine.

Reporting. Physicians responsible for the care of HIV-infected women should report all patients prescribed antiretroviral therapy in pregnancy to the Antiretroviral Pregnancy Registry, which in Europe is managed by Glaxo Wellcome. In the UK, all pregnant HIV-infected women should be reported anonymously to the National Study of HIV in Pregnancy. This is coordinated through the Royal College of Obstetricians and Gynaecologists (see Appendix II).

Prophylaxis and therapy for *Pneumocystis carinii* pneumonia. The mortality rate from a first infection with PCP is 5–20% in non-pregnant women, and is probably higher during pregnancy.

As in non-pregnant individuals, prophylaxis against PCP should be started when the CD4 count falls below 200/mm^3 or where there is a history of previous PCP infection. The preferred regimen is oral co-trimoxazole, which has been used for many years without reported teratogenicity. However, the constituent drugs do cross the placenta, and congenital malformations have been reported in animal models. Co-trimoxazole is a folate antagonist, and folate supplements should be prescribed. There is a theoretical risk of hemolysis and kernicterus in neonates following the use of sulfonamides in pregnancy, but there have been no reports of these conditions following maternal sulfamethoxazole therapy. When indicated, therefore, co-trimoxazole should be prescribed in pregnancy, in conjunction with folate supplements, as the adverse effects to the fetus are theoretical, in contrast to the known acute dangers of PCP for the mother.

Adverse reactions to co-trimoxazole are relatively frequent, and most commonly constitute a mild transient pruritus, abnormal liver function tests or megaloblastic anemia. However, severe reactions, including the potentially life-threatening Stevens–Johnson syndrome, may also occur.

In women who are allergic to co-trimoxazole, monthly inhalation of nebulized pentamidine isethionate should be administered. This has a low rate of systemic absorption and there have been no reports of teratogenesis. The combination of dapsone and pyrimethamine, although commonly used as an alternative form of prophylaxis in non-pregnant women, is best avoided antenatally as there is minimal experience of its use during pregnancy.

Effect of maternal HIV infection on pregnancy outcome

Studies from developing countries have demonstrated an increased risk of fetal loss, intrauterine growth retardation, preterm birth and low birthweight in women with HIV infection, irrespective of whether vertical transmission occurs. In industrialized countries, maternal HIV infection has been associated with an increased risk of first trimester miscarriage, but the course of pregnancy is otherwise unaffected unless the mother has advanced HIV disease. There is no increased risk of congenital abnormalities.

There has been concern that concurrent infection, notably with *Toxoplasma gondii*, cytomegalovirus and HSV, may adversely affect pregnancy outcome. Congenital toxoplasmosis may occur following reactivation of latent infection during pregnancy in HIV-positive women. Recent evidence suggests that the risk of congenital infection with *T. gondii* is very small, and is limited to those with CD4-positive lymphocyte counts below 200/mm^3. Infection with HSV type 2 (HSV-2) during pregnancy is more common in HIV-positive women, who are more prone to severe, prolonged episodes of all recurrent infections, including disseminated HSV. The risk of neonatal herpes does not appear to be increased, but whether HSV reactivation at delivery enhances perinatal HIV transmission is unclear.

Mother-to-child transmission of HIV

Mother-to-child transmission may occur *in utero*, intrapartum or postnatally through breastfeeding, and HIV has been demonstrated in fetal tissues during each trimester. Interventions to reduce the risk of mother-to-child transmission of HIV are shown in Table 4.5. In 1992, Bryson *et al.* proposed that, in the absence of breastfeeding:

- intrauterine infection should be presumed if an infected infant has HIV detectable by PCR or culture within 48 hours of birth
- intrapartum infection be presumed if an infected child had negative diagnostic tests (PCR, viral culture, p24Ag assays) during the first week of life, but these became positive within the next 3 months.

Based on these data, modeling analyses suggest that, in the absence of breastfeeding, around 65% of vertically infected infants acquire their infection during birth and approximately 35% are infected late *in utero* (within the last 2 months of pregnancy). Fewer than 2% are thought to

TABLE 4.5

Interventions to reduce the risk of mother-to-child HIV transmission

Intervention	Risk of mother-to-child transmission (%)
None	20–30
No breastfeeding	14–15
Zidovudine prophylaxis and no breastfeeding	5
Zidovudine prophylaxis, no breastfeeding and elective cesarean section	~2
Highly active antiretroviral therapy +/− elective cesarean section	< 2

be infected in the early and middle stages of pregnancy. These analyses are substantiated by a number of reports and observational studies; a study of HIV-infected pregnant women found that only 2% of fetuses aborted in the second trimester were HIV positive, and studies have demonstrated a greater risk of vertical transmission in first- rather than second-born twins. Moreover, there is no evidence for an HIV-associated congenital syndrome, HIV-infected and -uninfected babies are of similar birthweights, and HIV is undetectable at birth in approximately 70% of HIV-infected infants.

It is estimated that the mother-to-child HIV transmission rate ranges from 15 to 20% among non-breastfeeding European women to between 20 and 40% in breastfeeding African women. Risk for a particular individual or population depends on maternal, fetoplacental, intrapartum and postpartum factors (Table 4.6).

Maternal factors. It is well established that advanced maternal HIV disease, low antenatal CD4 counts and high mean maternal plasma viral loads are associated with an increased risk of vertical transmission. The latter is now recognized as the strongest predictor of vertical transmission.

Fetal factors. Infants who are born prematurely, or who are of low birthweight or small for gestational age are more likely to be infected with

TABLE 4.6

Factors associated with an increased risk of mother-to-child HIV transmission

- Maternal plasma viral load
- Severity of maternal HIV disease
- Preterm birth
- Prolonged rupture of the membranes
- Chorioamnionitis
- Vaginal delivery
- Breastfeeding

HIV. Whether this is a consequence of intrauterine infection or whether these infants are more susceptible to intrapartum infection is unclear. However, the evidence for higher intrapartum transmission rates would support the latter hypothesis. Pre-term infants may be more vulnerable to HIV transmission because of immature immune function, incompetent mucosal barriers or reduced levels of acquired maternal antibody. Active transport of maternal antibodies, which may protect the infant, occurs late in pregnancy.

Intrauterine factors. *In-utero* HIV infection occurs when the virus gains access to the fetus through the villous stroma and enters the fetal circulation, either by infection of the Hofbauer cells or by direct invasion of the syncytiotrophoblastic layer (Figure 4.1). The placenta and the fetal membranes are thought to protect the fetus from infection during pregnancy, and *in-utero* infection may result from a breach in these barriers. Prolonged rupture of the membranes is a well-established risk factor for vertical transmission; risk of transmission doubles if the membranes are ruptured for more than 4 hours.

Bacterial chorioamnionitis increases the risk of vertical transmission, and case reports have suggested amniocentesis as an iatrogenic cause of HIV transmission. Systemic infection with malaria or toxoplasma, placental abruption and cocaine misuse may cause placental damage and increase the risk of *in-utero* transmission.

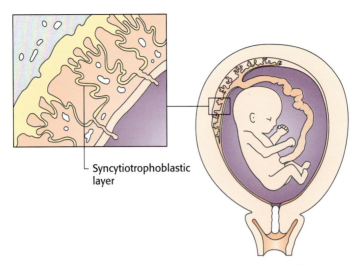

Syncytiotrophoblastic
layer

Figure 4.1 The HIV virus may gain access to the fetus through the villous stroma and enter the fetal circulation either by infection of the Hofbauer cells or by direct invasion of the syncytiotrophoblastic layer.

Intrapartum factors. HIV transmission most commonly occurs during labor and delivery, and there are two mechanisms by which this may occur. First, transmission may occur as a result of direct contact between the baby and infected blood and secretions within the female genital tract, through oro-mucosal exposure. Alternatively, transmission may result from maternal microtransfusions of blood entering the fetal circulation due to the force of contractions during labor and/or the presence of small areas of placental rupture. However, there is increasing evidence to support the former hypothesis. First, membrane rupture for greater than 4 hours increases the risk of vertical transmission. Second, at twin deliveries, the first-born twin has twice the risk of HIV infection compared with the second twin if both are delivered vaginally.

Conditions that predispose to increased shedding of HIV in the cervicovaginal secretions have been implicated as risk factors for vertical transmission. Most studies have demonstrated a correlation between maternal plasma viral load and detection of virus in cervicovaginal secretions, which may explain the increased rate of mother-to-child transmission in women with advanced HIV disease. No study to date has demonstrated a link between maternal STI status and vertical transmission, but a large observational study from Malawi has shown an association between maternal bacterial vaginosis and vertical transmission.

There have been case reports suggesting an association between blood-exposure events, such as the use of fetal scalp electrodes, placental abruption, episiotomy or lacerations, and vertical transmission, whereas others have not. It is probable that these factors are only weakly associated with HIV transmission.

Postnatal factors. Breastfeeding increases the background mother-to-child transmission rate by 14% in women infected with HIV before or during pregnancy, and by approximately 30% in women infected postnatally. It is well established that in developed countries, all HIV-infected women should be advised not to breastfeed.

Antiretroviral prophylaxis. The role of antiretroviral therapy in the prevention of mother-to-child transmission was first demonstrated in the AIDS Clinical Trial Group 076 (ACTG 076) trial, which was a multicenter, double-blind, placebo-controlled study involving women with CD4 counts above 200×10^6/liter. The majority of the women were asymptomatic and only 5% had received prior zidovudine therapy. Zidovudine was administered orally after the first trimester of pregnancy, intravenously during labor and delivery, and orally to the infant for the first 6 weeks of life. The trial demonstrated a two-thirds reduction in transmission from 22.6% in the placebo arm to 7.6% in the zidovudine arm.

A second perinatal-transmission study, ACTG 185, demonstrated a lower overall vertical transmission rate of 4.8% in those receiving the three-part zidovudine prophylaxis regimen. Moreover, the transmission rate in those with CD4 counts above 200/mm^3 was 3%, and there were no cases of mother-to-child transmission among the 48 women who had plasma viral load measurements below 500 copies/ml at delivery.

The mechanism by which zidovudine reduces vertical transmission is thought to involve both a reduction in plasma viral load and direct prophylaxis of the fetus and neonate. The optimum time to start zidovudine and the relative importance of the antepartum, intrapartum and neonatal components of the ACTG 076 regimen remain uncertain. Data from studies in Thailand, Burkino Faso and Côte d'Ivoire suggest that zidovudine prophylaxis started as late as the 36th week of pregnancy is beneficial. Data also exist which suggest that postnatal treatment alone provides a degree of protection from mother-to-child transmission.

The use of HAART regimens has become the standard of care for non-pregnant HIV-positive individuals requiring treatment. UK guidelines recommend that pregnancy *per se* should not preclude the use of such combination regimens where indicated for the health of the mother but that where possible, zidovudine should be one of the drugs used. Although there are few data on their efficacy in pregnancy, increasing numbers of observational studies are reporting little or no transmission in women taking combination therapy, even when the baby is delivered vaginally.

Recommendations. All pregnant HIV-positive women should be offered antiretroviral therapy to prevent perinatal transmission. For pregnant women in whom antiretroviral therapy is used solely to prevent mother-to-child transmission (i.e. those with low plasma viral loads and high CD4 counts), zidovudine monotherapy according to a modified version of the ACTG 076 regimen is currently recommended (Table 4.7). Therapy should be started at the beginning of the third trimester, and neonatal prophylaxis given for the first 3–6 weeks of life. Although the current consensus is that

TABLE 4.7

Zidovudine monotherapy for the prevention of mother-to-child transmission*

Stage	Dose	Timing
Antenatal	250 mg twice daily	From beginning of third trimester (around 29 weeks gestation)
Intrapartum	Loading dose: 2 mg/kg over 1 hour, followed by maintenance dose of 1 mg/kg hourly	From 1 hour prior to start of cesarean section (or at onset of labor) until umbilical cord clamped
Neonatal	2 mg/kg four times daily	For first 3–6 weeks of life

*From Taylor GP *et al.* 1999

antiretroviral therapy for non-pregnant adults should be initiated with three drugs (HAART), and that single-drug regimens are no longer justified, zidovudine monotherapy remains the only regimen for which substantial safety and efficacy data in pregnancy exist.

For those requiring antiretroviral therapy for maternal indications (i.e. those with high plasma viral loads and low CD4 counts), UK and North American guidelines recommend the use of HAART, in accordance with the standard of care for non-pregnant women (see pages 14–15).

Safety. More data are available on the safety in pregnancy of zidovudine than for any other antiretroviral agent. Among the children born to women participating in the first trial of zidovudine in pregnancy (ACTG 076), mild self-limiting anemia was the only complication seen in the zidovudine-exposed neonates, and there was no attributable adverse effects in the medium term (mean follow up 4.2 years).

In France, among 1754 children exposed to zidovudine, with or without lamivudine, eight cases of mitochondrial dysfunction have been reported, including two deaths. No deaths attributable to mitochondrial dysfunction were found in a review of 23 758 children born to HIV-positive mothers in the USA, including 12 353 children exposed to antiretroviral therapy during the perinatal period. Although these data are insufficient to confirm or refute a causal relationship, they have highlighted the need for continuing surveillance of children exposed to these drugs *in utero*.

Physicians prescribing antiretroviral therapy to pregnant women should report these pregnancies to the Antiretroviral Pregnancy Registry, which in Europe is managed by Glaxo Wellcome. No increased risk of congenital malformation has been found for zidovudine, or zidovudine plus lamivudine. As previously mentioned, data are sparse for other antiretrovirals.

Mode of delivery. Evidence from a European randomized, controlled trial and a meta-analysis of 15 prospective studies has demonstrated that cesarean section performed prior to labor, when the membranes are intact, reduces the risk of mother-to-child transmission by at least 50%. In non-breastfeeding women, receiving three-part zidovudine prophylaxis, whose babies are delivered in this way, the risk of transmission is approximately

2%. However, there are at present insufficient data to determine whether elective cesarean section confers any additional benefit in reducing transmission in women receiving HAART.

The vertical transmission risk for non-breastfeeding women with undetectable viral loads (less than 50 copies/ml) at the time of delivery is probably less than 2% irrespective of the mode of delivery. These women, particularly if they are multiparous with good obstetric histories, may consider vaginal delivery to be a relatively 'safe' option, in terms of vertical transmission risk. Women must be given sufficient information to allow an informed decision to be made regarding mode of delivery. Clear instructions should be written in the patient's notes concerning the need for intravenous zidovudine during labor and at delivery, and for a pediatrician to be present to assess the neonate and instigate zidovudine therapy.

Cesarean section. The benefits of cesarean section in reducing the risk of vertical transmission must be weighed against the possible risks. This mode of delivery carries a risk of anesthetic, intraoperative and postoperative complications, including hemorrhage, thromboembolism and infection. Whether these risks are greater in those with HIV infection is controversial but early reports suggesting that HIV disease is associated with impaired wound-healing and sepsis have not been substantiated. Women choosing a cesarean delivery should be strongly advised to have regional rather than general anesthesia, and the procedure should be carried out at around 38 weeks. All women should receive antibiotic prophylaxis. A zidovudine infusion should be started 1 hour before the start of the cesarean section, and should continue until the umbilical cord is clamped.

'Bloodless' cesarean section. A technique of 'bloodless' cesarean section has been advocated for HIV-positive women (Figure 4.2). A video of this procedure, including techniques of universal precaution in the operating room, is available (see Appendix II).

Vaginal delivery. It is vital that women choosing to deliver vaginally receive a zidovudine infusion at the onset of labor. For this reason, some obstetricians advocate that multiparous women, who are likely to have relatively quick and uncomplicated labors, should be admitted for induction of labor at around 38 weeks. Induction should be performed using prostaglandin gel rather than amniotomy. The use of invasive procedures during labor, such as fetal scalp electrodes and fetal blood sampling, should

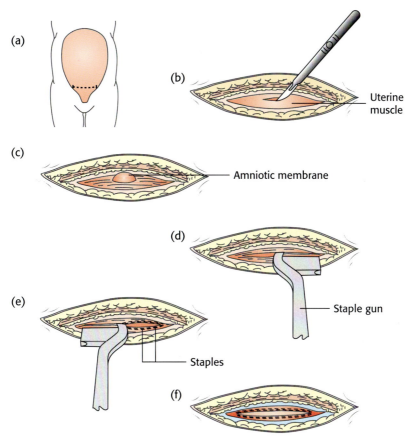

Figure 4.2 'Bloodless' cesarean section. (a) Routine abdominal entry incision including deflection of the bladder is performed. (b) Instead of opening the uterus using a large transverse incision with a scalpel, a small incision of approximately 1–2 cm in length, to the depth of the amniotic membranes, is made. Care should be taken to avoid rupture. (c) A small bleb of membrane emerges and a finger is inserted along the inside of the uterine muscle between the uterus and membranes. (d) A staple gun is inserted and, after checking to ensure that no parts of the fetus will be damaged, a row of absorbable staples are fired. These simultaneously give hemostasis and cut. (e) This procedure is then repeated in the opposite direction.
(f) The result is a standard-size opening in the uterus with complete hemostasis. Gloves should then be washed and any remaining blood in the abdomen removed using a Yank sucker. An incision is made in the amniotic membranes and the baby delivered without any contact with maternal blood.

45

be avoided. The membranes should be left intact for as long as possible, thus protecting the baby from prolonged contact with the maternal cervicovaginal secretions.

Emergency cesarean section should be performed for the usual obstetric reasons, and to avoid prolonged rupture of the membranes or a vaginal delivery that is likely to be difficult or prolonged. Where possible, trauma to the perineum by episiotomy or laceration should be avoided, as should delivery by vacuum extraction or forceps, which may cause fetal scalp abrasions. The zidovudine infusion should be discontinued when the umbilical cord is clamped. The third stage of labor should be actively managed to minimize the risk of postpartum hemorrhage.

Postnatal care

Mothers taking oral zidovudine prophylaxis should discontinue therapy after the delivery. However, those receiving combination regimens should continue their treatment. Adherence to combination regimens is particularly difficult in the postnatal period. The importance of not breastfeeding should be reiterated. Support and advice regarding formula feeding is vital.

In the developing world, malnutrition and infectious diseases are the primary causes of infant mortality. The benefit of breastfeeding in protecting against childhood infections needs to be balanced against the risks of increased childhood mortality associated with HIV acquisition through breast milk. Each country needs to assess its own perinatal mortality statistics, and adopt local guidelines regarding breastfeeding according to the resources available.

Care of the infant

After delivery, the umbilical cord is clamped and the baby washed and dried as soon as possible. Early cord clamping may reduce the risk of maternal cells entering the fetal circulation as the placenta detaches, and early cleansing and drying also reduce the chances of maternal secretions being ingested. Oral zidovudine should be administered to the infant for the first 3–6 weeks of life, and co-trimoxazole started thereafter until at least 6 months of age. Avoiding concurrent zidovudine and co-trimoxazole therapy reduces the risk of bone-marrow toxicity, as both these drugs are associated with bone-marrow suppression.

Diagnosis of infant infection

Maternal HIV antibodies cross the placenta and are detectable in most neonates of HIV-positive mothers. PCR (see page 12) is therefore used for the diagnosis of infant infections. A PCR test is carried out at birth, then at 3 weeks, 2 months and 6 months. For non-breastfed babies, over 90% of infants testing negative at 3 weeks of age and over 99% testing negative at 6 months of age will be uninfected. The definitive test is the HIV-antibody test; a negative result at 18 months confirms that the child is uninfected.

CHAPTER 5

Infection control

Patient-to-healthcare worker infection

Healthcare workers have a low but measurable risk of acquiring HIV infection following accidental exposure to infected blood or body fluids. Such occupational exposures include splash contamination (contact with the eyes, mouth or other mucous membranes), and percutaneous exposure, usually occurring as a result of a needlestick injury. Of the 52 healthcare workers with confirmed occupationally acquired HIV infection in the USA, the vast majority of transmissions involved blood or blood-stained body fluids; only three were laboratory workers exposed to HIV viral cultures. There have been no seroconversions as a result of injury from solid-bore needles. Nurses are the professional group at greatest risk, and there have been no confirmed seroconversions among surgeons.

Needlestick injury. The average risk of acquiring HIV infection after a single percutaneous exposure is 0.3%, which is substantially lower than the 30% and 3% risk for hepatitis B and hepatitis C viruses (HBV and HCV), respectively. Risk factors for seroconversion following needlestick exposure include deep injury, visible blood on the needle, needle placement in a vein or artery, and a source patient with high plasma viral load.

Splash contamination. The risk of seroconversion from mucosal surface exposure to an HIV-infected source is estimated at 0.09%. Large volumes of blood, prolonged duration of contact and a potential portal site of entry have been described as risk factors for transmission through splash contamination.

Post-exposure management. Regardless of actual risk, the psychological effect on a healthcare worker apparently exposed to HIV is substantial, particularly as he or she has to wait for 3 months before having an HIV test. During this time, they must avoid unprotected sex. It is also advisable to take a blood sample from the worker at the time of the needlestick injury. Analysis of this sample will confirm, if necessary, whether the worker was infected before the needlestick injury or whether infection was the result of occupational exposure. Such evidence is likely to improve prospects for compensation, although HIV infection has recently been recognized as an occupational illness for healthcare workers.

New regimens now exist that should be offered to healthcare workers following needlestick injury from known or suspected HIV-infected patients (Table 5.1).

Preoperative screening of patients has been suggested as a method of determining infection-control policy. This inevitably leads to a 'two-tier' infection control policy, in which women shown to be at risk are treated with great care, and those perceived as not being at risk are treated with less caution making cross-contamination more likely. In addition, a very small proportion of patients with primary HIV infection will be highly infectious, but will test negative.

When recommending infection-control policies, it is important to remember the problems associated with control of viral hepatitis. The risk of acquiring HBV and HCV infection is far greater than the risk of acquiring HIV infection, and yet it is not possible to select out patients carrying these blood-borne pathogens by patient-risk assessment. It has also proved impractical to screen for HBV and HCV prior to each operative intervention.

The small but measurable risk of occupationally acquired HIV infection coupled with the efficacy of post-exposure prophylaxis has reopened the debate on whether to test patients in order to protect the healthcare worker. Screening should not, however, reduce the pressure on healthcare workers to practise universal precautions – prevention almost invariably being better than cure.

Healthcare worker-to-patient infection

There has been only one recorded case of HIV transmission from a surgeon to a patient – namely that involving a dental surgeon in Florida. There were, however, a number of unusual features surrounding this case, including poor sterilization techniques and the possibility that contamination was

TABLE 5.1

CDC-recommended regimens for prophylaxis following occupational exposure to HIV

Type of exposure	Source material
Percutaneous	• Blood**
	– highest risk
	– increased risk
	– no increased risk
	• Fluid containing visible blood, other potentially infectious fluid† or tissue
	• Other body fluid, e.g. urine
Mucous membrane	• Blood
	• Fluid containing visible blood, other potentially infectious fluid† or tissue
	• Other body fluid, e.g. urine
Skin increased risk‡	• Blood
	• Fluid containing visible blood, other potentially infectious fluid† or tissue
	• Other body fluid, e.g. urine

*Four-week regimen is shown: zidovudine 250 mg, twice daily; lamivudine 150 mg, twice daily; indinavir 800 mg, three times daily
Highest risk – large volume of blood **and blood containing a high titer of HIV; increased risk – large volume of blood **or** blood containing a high titer of HIV; no increased risk – neither large volume of blood **nor** blood containing a high titer of HIV

deliberate. A high degree of public anxiety has been generated and on several occasions the press has called for compulsory screening of surgeons and healthcare professionals; this has not taken place.

In reality, patients are probably at greater risk of HBV and HCV infection from their surgeons than HIV infection. This raises the question of what to screen for and, subsequently, how often to test. As screening is unlikely to be either cost-effective or practical, the solution is to practise universal infection-control precautions.

A surgeon who thinks that he or she may have contracted a blood-borne pathogen has a duty to seek medical advice and a legal obligation to avoid

Prophylaxis	Antiretroviral regimen*
Recommend	Zidovudine plus lamivudine plus indinavir
Recommend	Zidovudine plus lamivudine, ± indinavir
Offer	Zidovudine plus lamivudine
Offer	Zidovudine plus lamivudine
Do not offer	
Offer	Zidovudine plus lamivudine, ± indinavir
Offer	
Do not offer	Zidovudine ± lamivudine
Offer	Zidovudine plus lamivudine, ± indinavir
Offer	Zidovudine ± indinavir
Do not offer	

†Includes semen, vaginal secretions, and cerebrospinal, synovial, pleural, peritoneal, pericardial and amniotic fluids
‡Exposures involving a high titer of HIV, prolonged contact, an extensive area, or an area in which skin integrity is visibly compromised; for skin exposures without increased risk, the risk from drug toxicity outweighs the benefits of prophylaxis

any invasive techniques that may place patients at risk. Failure to take these steps may result in criminal prosecution.

Infection-control precautions

The authors practise and endorse a policy of universal precautions for the purpose of infection control (Table 5.2).

In the operating room, gloves, masks, waterproof gowns and simple spectacles must be worn by the entire team. In addition, double gloving has been shown to result in a six-fold reduction in the rate of inner glove puncture. It is, however, impractical during longer procedures, and the

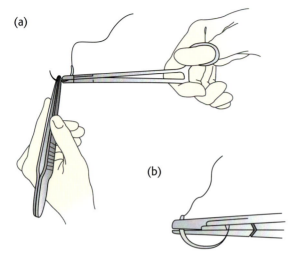

Figure 5.1 (a) The Smith safety needle holder has been designed to reduce the incidence of needlestick injury during surgery. (b) 'Parked' needle prior to knot tying or returning to the 'scrub nurse'.

authors recommend the use of blunt-tipped needles, which are associated with a reduction in the rate of glove puncture. They are suitable for all tissues except bladder and skin. The use of staples in skin is also part of the authors' recommended universal precautions. In addition, the authors

TABLE 5.2

Universal precautions for infection control against blood-borne pathogens

Use

- 'Sharp' boxes should be kept beside every hospital bed and not overfilled
- 'No touch' venesection
- Blunt-tipped needles
- Safety needle holders
- A magnet for picking up dropped sharps in theatre

Wear

- Waterproof gowns
- Spectacles
- Gloves

recommend using a new safety needle holder (Figure 5.1), which protects the sharp point of the needle, when knot tying and passing the used needle back to the 'scrub nurse'.

The precautions discussed are simple, relatively inexpensive to adopt and do not add additional operating time. They also have the capacity to reassure both staff and patient alike. A video showing techniques of universal precaution in the operating room is available (see Appendix II).

CHAPTER 6

Future trends

Prevention of sexual transmission of HIV infection

The starting point in the prevention of mother-to-child transmission of HIV infection must be the protection of women from sexually acquired HIV infection. For this reason, efforts must continue to promote changes in sexual behavior and the use of condoms. However, in developing countries, there is an urgent need for cheap alternative forms of HIV prevention that women themselves can control. The development of vaginal microbicidal agents may represent one such form of prevention, and these would be of particular value in countries where women may be unable to negotiate the use of condoms by their male partners.

Advances in therapy

The availability of combination antiretroviral therapy in industrialized countries has resulted in an increased life expectancy. However, earlier enthusiasm has been tempered with a greater awareness of adverse effects, the difficulties that patients have in adhering to drug regimens, and resulting drug resistance. Newer regimens necessitating less frequent dosing schedules with fewer tablets are likely to improve patient adherence and reduce the risk of drug resistance.

Reduction in mother-to-child transmission of HIV

A better understanding of measures that can reduce the risk of vertical transmission has led to a reduction in the number of babies born to women known to be HIV positive during pregnancy. However, in the UK the majority of pregnant HIV-positive women are not identified through antenatal testing. This deficiency is currently being addressed and the planned policy of non-coercive universal antenatal HIV testing should result in a fall in incidence of childhood HIV infection, in keeping with the USA and other western European countries. Combination antiretroviral regimens are cautiously being introduced into obstetric practice, and may further reduce the vertical transmission rate in developed countries, perhaps negating the benefits of elective cesarean section. Increasing numbers of women are conceiving while taking these combination regimens. More information regarding potential teratogenic and carcinogenic effects are awaited.

Short-course zidovudine prophylaxis during pregnancy, shown to be of benefit in recent studies from developing countries, may represent a cheaper, more feasible way of reducing the rate of vertical transmission in some resource-poor settings. Birth-canal washing with vaginal microbicidal agents represents a potential alternative intervention that does not require knowledge of the woman's HIV status and avoids the costs associated with HIV tests. However, an effective agent has not yet been developed.

Fertility

Life expectancy for people with HIV infection has improved significantly over recent years. Increasingly, couples where one or both individuals are HIV positive are requesting investigations and treatment for infertility. Cases should be assessed individually, with the involvement of local ethics committees. Data on the effectiveness of sperm-washing in reducing the risk of male-to-female transmission of HIV suggest that this technique is likely to become more widely available in the future.

Infection control

Infection-control procedures are improving all the time, and the current practice of universal precautions serves to protect healthcare workers from HIV and other blood-borne pathogens. New instrumentation in the surgical field will undoubtedly improve things further. Recent developments in terms of post-exposure prophylaxis are welcome.

Appendix I: Dosing and adverse effects of antiretroviral drugs

Drug	Dosing	Adverse effects
Nucleoside analogs		
Abacavir	300 mg twice daily	• Hypersensitivity reactions • Stevens–Johnson syndrome • Nausea • Diarrhea
Didanosine	400 mg once daily on empty stomach (lower doses if weight < 60 kg)	• Nausea • Bloating • Pancreatitis • Raised amylase • Peripheral neuropathy • Raised liver enzyme activity
Lamivudine	150 mg twice daily	• Nausea • Neutropenia • Anemia (rare) • Hair loss
Stavudine	40 mg twice daily (lower doses if weight < 60 kg)	• Peripheral neuropathy • Pancreatitis • Nausea • Raised liver enzyme activity
Zalcitabine	0.75 mg three times daily	• Peripheral neuropathy • Pancreatitis • Lactic acidosis and hepatic steatosis • Nausea
Zidovudine	250–300 mg twice daily	• Initial nausea • Bone-marrow suppression (5%) • Myopathy
Non-nucleoside reverse transcriptase inhibitors		
Nevirapine	200 mg twice daily (initially 200 mg once daily for 14 days)	• Rash • Stevens–Johnson syndrome • Raised liver enzyme activity

Delavirdine*	400 mg three times daily	• Rash • Stevens–Johnson syndrome
Efavirenz	600 mg once daily	• Rash • Dizziness • Headache • Insomnia • Vivid dreams • Raised liver enzyme activity • Reproductive toxicity in animal models, therefore contraindicated in women at risk of pregnancy

Protease inhibitors

Amprenavir	1200 mg twice daily	• Rash • Nausea • Diarrhea • Lipodystrophy • Peri-oral paresthesias
Indinavir	800 mg three times daily** (additional 1.5 liter fluid intake recommended)	• Nausea • Nephrolithiasis • Hyperbilirubinemia • Lipodystrophy
Nelfinavir	750 mg three times daily	• Diarrhea • Nausea
Ritonavir	600 mg twice daily** with dose escalation over 10–14 days	• Nausea • Vomiting • Diarrhea • Lipodystrophy • Peri-oral paresthesias • Raised liver enzyme activity • Raised lipids
Saquinavir soft-gel capsules	1200 mg three times daily**	• Nausea • Diarrhea • Lipodystrophy

*Not licensed in Europe

**Reduced dose when used in combination with other antiretroviral drugs

Appendix II: Addresses

Antiretroviral Pregnancy Registry

Physicians responsible for the care of HIV-infected women should report all patients prescribed antiretroviral therapy in pregnancy to:

In the USA

Antiretroviral Pregnancy Registry, PO Box 13398, Glaxo Wellcome, Research Triangle Park, NC 27709-3398
Tel: 919 483 9437
Fax: 919 315 8981

In the UK

National Study of HIV in Pregnancy, Royal College of Obstetricians and Gynaecologists, 27 Sussex Place, Regent's Park, London NW4 RG1
Tel: 020 7829 8686

Antiretroviral Pregnancy Registry, International Product Safety and Pharmacovigilance, Glaxo Wellcome Research and Development, Greenford Road, Greenford, Middlesex UB6 0HE
Tel: 020 8422 3434

Video

The video referred to on pages 44 and 53 is available from:
The TV Unit, Charing Cross Hospital, Fulham Palace Road, London W6 8RF, UK

Key references

HIV INFECTION

Mastro TD, de Vincenzi I. Probability of sexual HIV-1 transmission. *AIDS* 1996;10(suppl A):S75–82.

Pantaleo G, Graziosi C, Fauci AS. New concepts in the immunopathogenesis of human immunodeficiency virus infection. *N Engl J Med* 1993;328:327–35.

Quinn TC, Wawer MJ, Sewankambo N *et al.* Viral load and heterosexual transmission of human immunodeficiency virus type 1. Rakai Project Study Group. *N Engl J Med* 2000;342:921–9.

Smith JR, Kitchen VS. *Infection in Gynaecology.* Edinburgh: Churchill Livingstone, 1994.

MANAGING INFECTED WOMEN

British HIV Association (BHIVA) guidelines for the treatment of HIV-infected adults with antiretroviral therapy. Issued December 1999. (Guidelines updated and accessed via www.aidsmap.com)

Chin KM, Sidhu JS, Janssen RS *et al.* Invasive cervical cancer in human immunodeficiency virus-infected and uninfected hospital patients. *Obstet Gynecol* 1998;92:83–7.

Fontanet AL, Saba J, Chandelying V *et al.* Protection against sexually transmitted diseases by granting sex workers in Thailand the choice of using the male or female condom: results from a randomized controlled trial. *AIDS* 1998;12:1851–9.

Grosskurth H, Mosha F, Todd J *et al.* Impact of improved treatment of sexually transmitted diseases on HIV infection in rural Tanzania: a randomised controlled trial. *Lancet* 1995;346:530–6.

Kim LU, Johnson MR, Barton S *et al.* Evaluation of sperm washing as a potential method of reducing HIV transmission in HIV-discordant couples wishing to have children. *AIDS* 1999;13:645–51.

Safrin S, Grunfeld C. Fat distribution and metabolic changes in patients with HIV infection. *AIDS* 1999;13:2493–505.

Semprini AE, Fiore S, Pardi G. Reproductive counselling for HIV-discordant couples. *Lancet* 1997; 349:1401–2.

Shah PN, Smith JR, Wells C *et al.* Menstrual symptoms in women infected by the human immunodeficiency virus. *Obstet Gynecol* 1994;83:397–400.

Sinei SK, Morrison CS, Sekadde-Kigondu C *et al.* Complications of use of intrauterine devices among HIV-1-infected women. *Lancet* 1998;351:1238–41.

Six C, Heard I, Bergeron C *et al.* Comparative prevalence, incidence and short-term prognosis of cervical squamous intraepithelial lesions amongst HIV-positive and HIV-negative women. *AIDS* 1998;12:1047–56.

Vernon SD, Holmes KK, Reeves WC. Human papillomavirus infection and associated disease in persons infected with human immunodeficiency virus. *Clin Infect Dis* 1995;suppl 1:S121–4.

OBSTETRIC CARE

Blanche S, Tardieu M, Rustin P *et al.* Persistent mitochondrial dysfunction and perinatal exposure to antiretroviral nucleoside analogues. *Lancet* 1999; 354:1084–9.

Brossard Y, Aubin JT, Mandelbrot L *et al.* Frequency of early in utero HIV-1 infection: a blind DNA polymerase chain reaction study on 100 fetal thymuses. *AIDS* 1995;4:359–66.

Bryson YJ, Luzuriaga K, Sullivan JL, Wara DW. Proposed definitions for in utero versus intrapartum transmission of HIV-1. *N Engl J Med* 1992;327:1246–7.

Connor EM, Sperling RS, Gelber R *et al.* Reduction of maternal-infant transmission of human immunodeficiency virus type 1 with zidovudine treatment. Pediatric AIDS Clinical Trials Group Protocol 076 Study Group. *N Engl J Med* 1994; 331:1173–80.

Duliege AM, Amos CI, Felton S *et al.* Birth order, delivery route, and concordance in the transmission of human immunodeficiency virus type 1 from mothers to twins. International Registry of HIV-Exposed Twins. *J Pediatr* 1995; 126:625–32.

Landesman SH, Kalish LA, Burns DN *et al.* Obstetrical factors and the transmission of human immunodeficiency virus type 1 from mother to child. The Women and Infants Transmission Study. *N Engl J Med* 1996;334:1617–23.

Mofenson LM, Lambert JS, Stiehm ER *et al.* Risk factors for perinatal transmission of human immunodeficiency virus type 1 in women treated with zidovudine. Pediatric AIDS Clinical Trials Group Study 185 Team. *N Engl J Med* 1999;341:385–93.

Taylor GP, Lyall H, Mercey D *et al.* British HIV Association guidelines for prescribing antiretroviral therapy in pregnancy (1998). *Sex Trans Infect* 1999;75:90–7.

The European Mode of Delivery Collaboration. Elective Caesarean-section versus vaginal delivery in prevention of vertical HIV-1 transmission: a randomised clinical trial. *Lancet* 1999;353:1035–9.

The International Perinatal HIV Group. The mode of delivery and the risk of vertical transmission of human immunodeficiency virus type 1: a meta-analysis of 15 prospective cohort studies. *N Engl J Med* 1999; 340:977–87.

Wabwire-Mangen F, Gray RH, Mmiro FA *et al.* Placental membrane inflammation and risks of maternal-to-child transmission of HIV-1 in Uganda. *J Acquir Immune Defic Syndr* 1999;22:379–85.

Wade NA, Birkhead GS, Warren BL. Abbreviated regimens of zidovudine prophylaxis and perinatal transmission of the human immunodeficiency virus. *N Engl J Med* 1998;339:1409–14.

INFECTION CONTROL

Reducing mother-to-child transmission of HIV infection in the United Kingdom. Recommendations of an intercollegiate working party for enhancing voluntary confidential HIV testing in pregnancy. London: Royal College of Paediatrics and Child Health, Royal College of Pathologists, Royal College of

Obstetricians and Gynaecologists, Public
Health Laboratory Service, Royal College
of Nursing, Royal College of General
Practitioners, Royal College of Midwives,
April 1998.

Stafford MK, Kitchen VS, Smith JR.
Reducing the risk of blood-borne infection
in surgical practice. *Br J Obstet Gynaecol*
1995;102:439–41.

FUTURE TRENDS

Gilling-Smith C, Smith JR, Semprini AE.
HIV and infertility: time to treat. *BMJ*
2001;322:566–7.

McCormack S, Hayes R, Lacey CJ *et al.*
Microbicides in HIV prevention. *BMJ*
2001;322:410–13.

Mofenson LM. Short-course zidovudine
for prevention of perinatal infection.
Lancet 1999;353:766–7.

Mofenson L, McIntyre JA. Advances and
research directions in the prevention of
mother-to-child HIV-1 transmission.
Lancet 2000;355:2237–44.

Further information is available at:

www.aidsmap.com (UK)
www.hivatis.org (USA)

Index